YOUR KNOWLEDGE HAS VALUE

AF156986

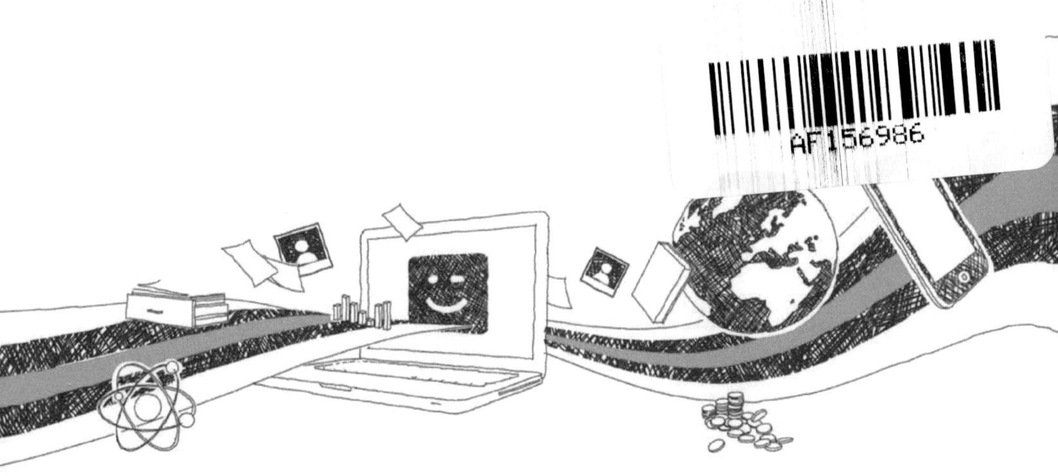

- We will publish your bachelor's and master's thesis, essays and papers
- Your own eBook and book - sold worldwide in all relevant shops
- Earn money with each sale

Upload your text at www.GRIN.com and publish for free

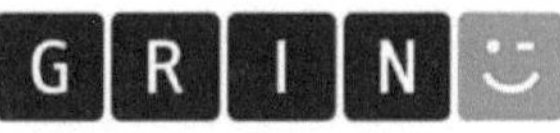

Bibliographic information published by the German National Library:

The German National Library lists this publication in the National Bibliography; detailed bibliographic data are available on the Internet at http://dnb.dnb.de .

This book is copyright material and must not be copied, reproduced, transferred, distributed, leased, licensed or publicly performed or used in any way except as specifically permitted in writing by the publishers, as allowed under the terms and conditions under which it was purchased or as strictly permitted by applicable copyright law. Any unauthorized distribution or use of this text may be a direct infringement of the author s and publisher s rights and those responsible may be liable in law accordingly.

Imprint:

Copyright © 1987 GRIN Verlag, Open Publishing GmbH
Print and binding: Books on Demand GmbH, Norderstedt Germany
ISBN: 9783668577497

This book at GRIN:

http://www.grin.com/en/e-book/381210/measurement-of-surface-tension-in-urines-of-495-out-patients-of-a-private

Hanspeter Moser

Measurement of Surface Tension in Urines of 495 Out-Patients of a Private Office

Urology

GRIN Publishing

GRIN - Your knowledge has value

Since its foundation in 1998, GRIN has specialized in publishing academic texts by students, college teachers and other academics as e-book and printed book. The website www.grin.com is an ideal platform for presenting term papers, final papers, scientific essays, dissertations and specialist books.

Visit us on the internet:

http://www.grin.com/

http://www.facebook.com/grincom

http://www.twitter.com/grin_com

Measurement of Surface Tension in Urines of 495 Out-Patients of a Private Office

PhD-Thesis
Department of Urology at Case Western Reserve University, Cleveland, Ohio, USA, Professor Elroy D. Kursh, M.D.

By
Dr. med. Hanspeter Moser, Eau-Board-certified Urologist
Isernhagen, Germany
Türkiskamp 9

Isernhagen, 4th of April, 1987

Acknowledgement

I am deeply grateful to Professor Dr. med. Hans-Joachim Merker, Director of the Anatomical Institute of the Free University Berlin for his initiation of this work. It was his question why human urine was sometimes foamy that started this investigation.

1. Introduction

Several proposals for methods to investigate the changes in the surface tension of biological or body fluids have been made already, since it has been suspected that such changes might reflect a pathophysiological status of the respective organism. Data on systematic measurements of the surface tension of various physiological fluids have been published, but not yet for urine during various urological diseases.

Measurements of the surface tension of amniotic fluid were carried out clinically in conjunction with the respiratory distress syndrome (6, 7, 9). Other measurements of the surface tension were performed on bile, blood, cerebrospinal fluid, serum, lymph, saliva and tears.

ABSOLOM et al. (1) investigated in 1983, whether substrates with different surface tensions would induce a different degree of conformational change in adsorbed protein molecules, and whether these differences in the degree of change would be reflected by differences in the surface tension of the adsorbed layers. Their results were in good agreement with the relative hydrophobicity of the investigated proteins, as determined by other, independent methods.

MYSELS (10) carried out surface tension studies of bile salts dissolved in water with the purpose to show that, on the base of certain assumptions, the results of measurements of the surface tension of the solution may be translatable directly into the monomer activity and thus yield an indication for correlation.

It is well known, that at any border surface between air and a liquid intermolecular forces of attraction become effective with the tendency to minimize the surface of the liquid. From measurements of the surface tension in alveoli it is e.g. known that the layer of liquid on the alveolar wall has to contain substances reducing the surface tension. Subxtances showing this property consist of molecules with strong mutual forces of attraction, but with low forces of attraction against the other molecules of the liquid. For this reason, such molecules accumulate at the surface of the liquid, reducing the surface tension. They are therefore also called "surface active substances" or "surfactants".

Some surface active substances have been successfully indentified chemically. The alveolar film of liquid e.g. contains a mixture of proteins and lipoids, with derivates of lecithin most likely determining the specific surface activity.

At the urothelium also, e.g. at least by means of a scanning electron microscope, a high membrane turnover can be demonstrated also (8). Accordingly the question arises, whether in various disorders, such as hyperuricemia, diabetes mellitus, chronical pyelonephritis, diathesis for calcium oxalate lithiasis, carcinomas of the urothelium etc. a change in the surface tension of the urine can be observed or not, as a differential test with respect to patients with e.g. lumbar symptoms.

Several methods exist for measuring the interfacial or the surface tension, respectively.

Physically the surface of a substance constitutes a special form of the border surface, i.e. the surface forms the border surface between gaseous and liquid phases of substances, while a border surface represents the area between two condensed phases of substances.

The surface tension is a physically measurable tensorial force, the molecules in the border region of the condensed phase of a liquid are exposed to. While the actual tensorial force cannot be measured directly, the resulting surface tension can be determined.

Methods based on measurement of a force are e.g. the ring method, by which the force required to pull a ring immersed into the liquid with a wetted circumference of defined length through the border surface is measured, or the plate method, using principally a similar approach, but not requiring hydrostatic corrections (12).

In France, the stirrup method, employing a length of wire stretched horizontally in a frame, has found some use.

Pressure measuring methods observe the rise of a liquid in capillaries or determine the maximum pressure in gas bubbles.

Optical methods generally are based on optical measuring of a distance or of an angle on a drop of the liquid. Common procedures are the so-called "Pending drop method" or the "Sessile drop method" and similar approaches.

2. Materials and methods

A tensiometer Model K 10 (Kruess Corp., 2000 Hamburg, Fed. Rep. Germany) based on the "Ring-method" was used for measuring the surface tension of the urine.

2.1. The Ring Method

A platinum ring suspended horizontally is immersed into the liquid and subsequently lifted out of the liquid again. By means of this method, the force K_{max} required to pull the ring with a wetted circumference of length L_b through the border surface is measured.

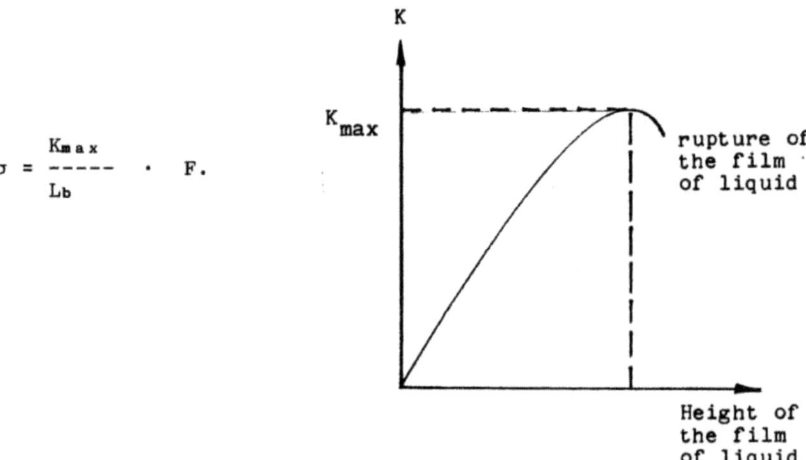

Fig.: The force acting on the ring as a function of the height of the film of liquid

The ring method was known in the past century already. Following the description of a "Ring-Tensiometer" by LECOMPTE DU NOÜY in 1919, the procedure became worldwide the preferred method. The principal advantages of the method are:

- simplicity of execution
- short measuring intervals
- high resolution of the measured values
- neglibility of the wetting angle
- availability of additional information from the shape of the "Film rupture characteristic".

All these facts are most likely the reason for the undiminished popularity and preferred use of the ring method.

A ring with geometrically precisely defined dimensions, made of PtIr 20 alloy and suspended horizontally, is used as the measuring probe.

The selection of the platinum-iridium alloy mentioned is based on the following properties:

- excellent wettability
- chemical inertness and stability
- high melting point
- considerably mechanical strength

The wetted length L_b ist determined by the geometrical configuration of the ring, characterized by the mean diameter 2 R of the ring and by the diameter 2 r of the wire the ring is made of.

The following dimensions of the ring have generally been accepted:

$$R = 9.545 \text{ mm}$$
$$r = 0.185 \text{ mm}$$
$$L_b = 119.95 \text{ mm}$$

These dimensions represent compromises between the demands for:

- high measuring accuracy (R as large as possible, r as small as possible)
- convenient size for easy handling
- good mechanical stability of the ring
- minimal quantity of liquid sample required (R as small as possible, r as large as possible)

The standard configuration of the ring as described requires the volume of the liquid sample to be at least 10 ml. Special rings offered by KRÜSS Corporation, Hamburg, Fed. Rep. of Germany, allow evaluation of samples with a volume as low as 0.2 ml with reduced accuracy. Stretching the method that far is particularly valuable in medical applications, where frequently samples of body fluids are obtainable in very limited quantities only.

2.2. Details of the measuring procedure

2.2.1. Border surface between a liquid and a gaseous phase

Preceding immersion, the force measuring system, including the horizontally suspended ring, is carefully tared.

The ring is subsequently immersed into the liquid to be investigated until completely wetted and subsequently lifted again until the force required to lift the ring has reached the maximum, respectively until rupture of the film of liquid occurs.

During the lifting procedure the surface tension acts along the wetted line on the ring, with the point of action migrating along the circumference of the wire forming the ring.

As illustrated in the figure, the resultant of the forces acting on the ring reaches a maximum for the tangents of the film of liquid on the circumference of the ring being perpendicular to the plane of the ring. This maximum is measured.

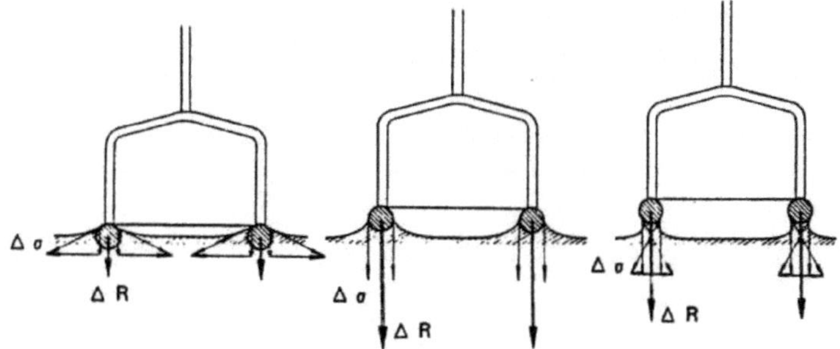

Contrary to the widespread opinion, it is therefore not necessary to lift the ring until rupture of the film of liquid occurs, to determine the surface tension of the liquid. Except for the hydrostatic correction required, the wetting angle is also primarily without an influence of the result of the measuring procedure.

2.2.2. Border surface between two liquid phases

Except for somewhat more elaborate preliminaries, the procedure for determination of the tension of the border surface between two liquid phases is similar to the measurement of the surface tension of a liquid.

In the course of the first step, the force measuring system is tared carefully with the ring completely immersed into the phase with lower specific gravity.

Subsequently a new beaker is approximately half filled with the phase with the higher specific gravity, the ring cleaned and immersed into that phase. A sufficient volume of the phase with lower specific gravity is then very carefully placed on top of the first phase. Measuring of the tension of the border surface between the two phases is then performed as described before by measuring the maximum of the force observed during lifting the ring out of the phase with the higher specific gravity.

Taring of the force measuring system with the ring immersed into the phase with the lower specific gravity serves for compensation of the buoyancy of the ring and of the surface tension acting on the vertical supports for the ring.

2.2.3. Evaluation of the results of the measurements

The results of the measurements are evaluated using the expression

$$\sigma = \frac{K_{max}}{L_b} \cdot F$$

where: σ = surface tension (mN/m)
K_{max} = maximum of the force (nM)
L_b = length of the ring wetted (m)
F = correction factor

L_b is known from the dimensions of the ring, while K_{max} is measured.

In addition to the resultant from the surface tension, the hydrostatic weight of the volume of liquid V_h below the ring lifted together with the ring is included in the result of the measurement. This additional force has to be eliminated by means of a correction factor.

To achieve the necessary stability, the ring also cannot comply with the theoretical requirement of

$$R/r \longrightarrow \infty$$

Consequently, during each measuring procedure, not only one, but two maxima of the force resulting from the surface tension are actually occuring, with the tangent of the surface of the outer film of liquid to the circumference being first perpendicular to the plane of the ring and then the tangent of the inner film of liquid. This detail is important for measurements calling for utmost precision only however.

In a paper publihed in 1930, HARKINS and JORDAN presented an extensive table of values for F determined empirically. The two scientists had noted similar geometrical shapes of the films of liquid to be associated with similar correction factors. It proved to be possible to describe the geometrical shapes by the dimensionless expressions

$$R^3 / V$$

and

$$R / v$$

with V representing the volume of liquid lifted by capillary action.

The table covers the ranges for

R^3 / V between 0.3 and 3.5

and

R / r between 30 and 60

Parallel to the work of HARKINS and JORDAN, theoretical determination of the shapes of the inner and outer meniscus (FREUD/FREUD) confirmed the correctness of the table and the error limit of 0.25 % only. The table of correction factors remains actual to the present day.

Modern tensiometers feature linear compensation, being adjusted to have a correction factor of unity for water at a temperature of 20 degrees centigrade.

Correction of values for the border surface tension measured is advantageously performed using the equation by ZIDEMA and WALTERS (1941) standardized by the American Society for Testing and Materials (ASTM):

$$F = 0.725 + \sqrt{\frac{0.01452 \cdot \sigma^*}{\frac{B_b{}^2}{4} \quad (D - d)} + 0.04534 - \frac{1.679}{R/r}}$$

where

D, d = specific gravity of the denser, resp. of the less dense liquid (g/cm^3)

σ^* = border surface tension measured (mN/m)

L_b = $4 \pi R^2$, wetted length of the ring (m)

2.2.4. Remarks concerning the measuring accuracy

The degree of accuracy obtainable using the ring method is primarily limited by the correction factor F, since physical determination of the geometrical configuration of the ring and measurement of the force incurred during lifting of the ring can be carried out with a five digit accuracy at least. Absolute precision down to less than 0.01 nM/m cannot be achieved in practice, while the results are quite reproducible down to 0.01 nM/m.

2.2.5. Measurement on solutions containing tensides

Measurements on solutions containing surface active molecules, such as tensides, pose special problems. As the name implies, surface active molecules aggregate at the border surfaces. Due to their bipolar characteristics they practically form an interface between the borders of the phases, resulting in lowering of the tension of the border surface, resp. of the surface.

Very small amounts of tensides are already capably of causing considerable effects. When measuring surface tension of such solutions, the time required for the process of aggregation of the tenside molecules constitutes the main problem. While for high concentrations of tensides equilibrium is reached within fractions of a second, depending on the chemical structure of the tenside molecules hours may be required for low concentrations. Accordingsly the surface tension may be dependent on the "age" of a surface itself.

If now new surfaces are formed during the measurement of the surface tension, as this is the case during lifting of the ring, the age of the surface composed of "old" peripheral areas and the "young" areas of the collar directly below the ring is no longer precisely defined.

In the practice of measurement, such conditions may cause controversial results - each new measurement at the same sample yielding a different value, which is mostly lower than the preceding result, quasi indicating some sort of "drift". Numerous investigators then questioned the correct operation of their measuring set-up. In such cases it is important not to disturb the order of the molecules at the border surface by avoiding rupture of the film of liquid after transgressing the maximum of the force encountered during lifting of the ring.

To bypass the problems described, an arrangement featured by the digital tensiometer made by KRÜSS Corp. in Hamburg, is particularly helpful: Following an automatic stop of the lift exactly in the point the maximum force and a subsequent minute lowering of the ring, the maximum can be tested again within a few seconds without significant formation of new surface. This provision permits reliable determination of an eventual drift in the results.

Concludingly it may be mentioned, that surface films exposed to repeated expansion and compression, such as this is the case during lifting and lowering of the ring, may influence the measured value in a fashion which frequently cannot be reproduced reliably.

2.3. Procedure

The fresh middle portion of the discharge of urine, or urine obtained by means of catheterization of a total of 495 patients of a urological practice with different disorders of the urinary tract. All patients (190 female, 305 male) were examined by means of infusion-urography, sonography and/or cystoscopy. In addition to the usual cytological investigations, the following serum parameters were determined: Level of uric acid, Level of urea, Level of creatinine, Blood count, Levels of Ca, Na and K in the serum, Level of parathormone in the serum (for patients suffering from calcium-oxalate-lithiasis).

The values for the surface tension of the urine obtained were classified according to the following criteria:

- Age of the patient
- Sex of the patient
- pH of the urine
- Sediments observed in the urine (according to BROSIG: Zentrifugation 5' with 1500 rounds/minute. Magnification 10 high-powered fields (400x) were counted.
- quantity of bacteria in urine (culture on Urotube, Fa. Roche, Basel, Switzerland. Infection: 10^5 - 10^7 counts)
- Urological disorders present
- Metabolic disorders present
- Missing urological disorders (Lumbar symptoms)
- Erythrocyte count in the urine
- Leucocyte count in the urine

The levels of uric acid, creatinine, Ca, Na and K and the others were determined in the urine.

Preceding each measurement, the measuring vessel was rinsed repeatedly with acetone and subsequently pulled through a flame.

Evaluation of the results was performed on a personal computer compatible with the AT series of computers made by IBM Corporation.

The results were entered into data acquisition forms designed for electronic data processing and initially acquired with the data bank system "d Base II +". Actual statistical evaluation was carried out using the program parcel "SPSS-PC +". Variance analysis and single and multifactorial regression procedures were employed. Group differences were declared to be significant for $p \leq 0.05$.

Results

Simple computation of the mean value for all 495 cases yielded a mean surface tension of 44.27 nM/m (SD 4.50). For women (n = 190) a mean value of 44.35 nM/m (SD 5.04) and for men (n = 305) a mean value of 44.22 nM/m (SD 4.15) was determined. No difference specific to sex exists therefore.

When classified according to the age of the patients, the values measured showed no remarkable differences either. Fig. 1 offers a review of the mean surface tension measured with respect to the age and the sex of the patients.

Statistics:

Table 1:

SEX and surface tension

Value Label	Sum	Mean	Std Dev	Sum of Sq	Cases
1 female	8426.7000	44.3511	5.0379	4796.8948	190
2 male	13487.1000	44.2200	4.1454	5223.9280	305
within Groups Total	21913.8000	44.2703	4.5085	10020.8228	495

Analysis of Variance

Source	Sum of Squares	D.F.	Mean Square	F	Sig.
Between Groups	2.0107	1	2.0107	.0989	0.7533
Within Groups	10020.8228	493	20.3262		

Eta = .0142 Eta Squared = .0002

Figure 1

Mean surface tension of urine given with respect to age and sex of 495 patients.

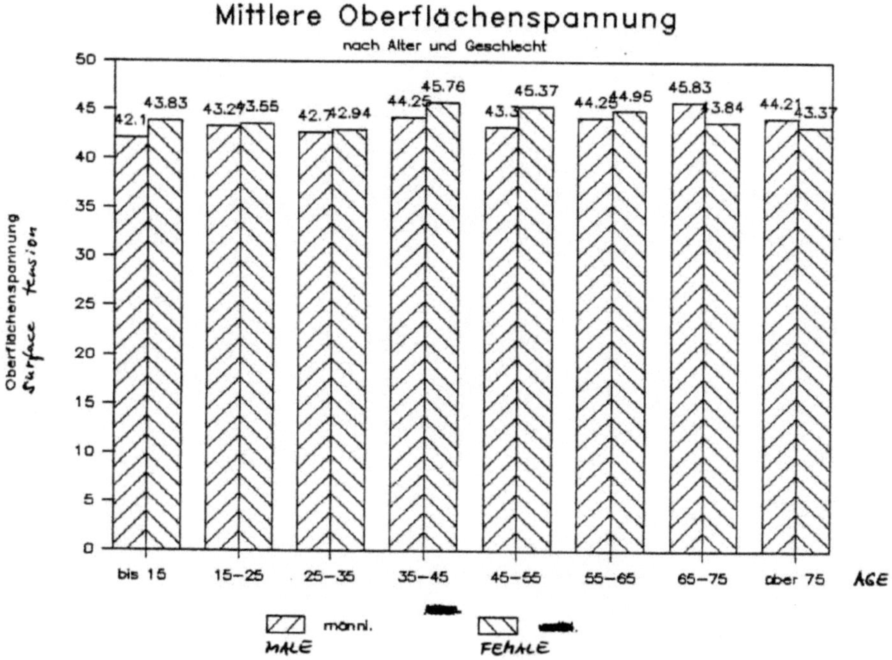

Evaluation by variance analysis with respect to the electrolyte levels (Figs. 2 through 4), the pH-value (Fig. 5) the level of uric acid (Fig. 6) and the level of ceatinine (Fig. 7) likewise yielded no significant group differences. See also tables No. 2 to No. 7.

Statistics:

Table 2:

Na^+ (urine) and surface tension

Value Label	Sum	Mean	Std Dev	Sum of Sq	Cases
1. - 40	2004.7000	43.5804	4.1008	756.7524	46
2. 40 - 80	3993.8000	45.3841	5.0820	2246.8977	88
3. 80 - 120	4974.8000	44.0248	4.6848	2458.0906	113
4. 120 - 160	5448.7000	44.6615	4.1576	2091.5489	122
5. 160 - 200	2989.3000	43.9603	4.0178	1081.5828	68
6. 200 - 240	1286.3000	42.8767	4.8053	669.6337	30
7. 240 - 280	512.1000	42.6750	3.7112	151.5025	12
8. 280 - 320	298.0000	42.5714	4.4414	118.3543	7
9. 320 -	346.1000	45.5125	4.7643	158.8887	8
within Groups Total	21871.8000	44.2749	4.4798	9733.2517	494

Analysis of Variance

Source	Sum of Squares	D.F.	Mean Square	F	Sig.
Between Groups	284.4171	8	35.5521	1.7715	0.0803
Within Groups	9733.2517	485	20.0686		

Eta = .1685 Eta Squared = .0284

Table 3:

Ca^{++} (urine) and surface tension

Value Label	Sum	Mean	Std Dev	Sum of Sq	Cases
1. - 2.5	4703.3000	44.7933	4.6288	2228.2853	105
2. 2.5 - 5.0	5750.8000	44.5798	5.0341	3241.4876	129
3. 5.0 - 7.5	4523.5000	43.9175	4.0759	1694.4885	103
4. 7.5 - 10.0	2340.3000	44.1566	4.2212	926.5702	53
5. 10.0 - 12.5	1700.0000	43.5897	3.6641	510.1759	39
6. 12.5 - 15.0	1193.0000	44.1852	4.4731	520.2141	27
7. 15.0 - 17.5	828.7000	43.6158	4.1801	314.5253	19
8. 17.5 - 20.0	358.9000	44.8625	5.4696	209.4188	8
9. 20.0 -	473.3000	43.0273	5.2127	271.7218	11
within Groups Total	21871.8000	44.2749	4.5219	9916.8875	494

Analysis of Variance

Source	Sum of Squares	D.F.	Mean Square	F	Sig.
Between Groups	100.7813	8	12.5977	.6161	0.7646
Within Groups	9916.8875	485	20.4472		

Eta = .1003 Eta Squared = .0101

Table 4:

K^+ (urine) and surface tension

Value Label	Sum	Mean	Std Dev	Sum of Sq	Cases
1. - 25	1809.6000	46.4000	4.7026	840.3400	39
2. 25 - 50	5837.6000	43.8917	4.9475	3231.0809	133
3. 50 - 75	6717.4000	44.1934	4.5988	3193.4534	152
4. 75 - 100	4073.5000	43.8011	4.1161	1558.6899	93
5. 100 - 125	2016.4000	44.8089	3.0845	418.6164	45
6. 125 - 150	708.1000	44.2563	4.3534	284.2794	16
7. 150 - 175	273.3000	45.5500	4.4769	100.2150	6
8. 175 -	435.9000	43.5900	4.0300	146.1690	10
within Groups Total	21871.8000	44.2749	4.4843	9772.8440	494

Analysis of Variance

Source	Sum of Squares	D.F.	Mean Square	F	Sig.
Between Groups	244.8247	7	34.9750	1.7393	0.0977
Within Groups	9772.8440	486	20.1087		

Eta = .1563 Eta Squared = .0244

Statistics:

Table 5:

urine - pH and surface tension

Value Label	Sum	Mean	Std Dev	Sum of Sq	Cases
1. 5.2	86.2000	43.1000	8.6267	74.4200	2
2. 5.5	1617.5000	43.7162	3.5597	456.1703	37
3. 5.8	2809.7000	44.5984	4.2639	1127.2298	63
4. 6.0	47.5000	47.5000	0.0	0.0	1
5. 6.2	9306.5000	43.8986	4.4827	4240.0096	212
6. 6.5	5890.1000	44.6220	4.8261	3051.1063	132
7. 6.6	47.0000	47.0000	0.0	0.0	1
8. 6.8	817.1000	45.3944	5.6007	533.2494	18
9. 7.0	134.0000	44.6667	2.4664	12.1667	3
10. 7.4	1070.2000	44.5917	4.2643	418.2383	24
within Groups Total	21825.8000	44.2714	4.5302	9912.5904	493

Analysis of Variance

Source	Sum of Squares	D.F.	Mean Square	F	Sig.
Between Groups	110.0763	9	12.2307	.5960	0.8007
Within Groups	9912.5904	483	20.5230		

Eta = .1048 Eta Squared = .0110

Table 6:

uric acid (urine) and surface tension

Value Label	Sum	Mean	Std Dev	Sum of Sq	Cases
1. - 15	1872.6000	44.5857	5.8250	1391.1514	42
2. 15 - 30	5882.6000	44.5652	4.9811	3250.2597	132
3. 30 - 45	8293.4000	44.1138	4.0141	3013.0840	188
4. 45 - 60	3816.3000	43.8655	4.4253	1684.1966	87
5. 60 - 75	1423.2000	44.4750	4.1774	540.9600	32
6. 75 - 90	311.3000	44.4714	1.7566	18.5143	7
7. 90 - 105	82.9000	41.4500	.6364	.4050	2
8. 105 -	189.5000	47.3750	3.0826	28.5075	4
within Groups Total	21871.8000	44.2749	4.5195	9927.0785	494

Analysis of Variance

Source	Sum of Squares	D.F.	Mean Square	F	Sig.
Between Groups	90.5902	7	12.9415	.6336	0.7282
Within Groups	9927.0785	486	20.4261		

Eta = .0951 Eta Squared = .0090

Table 7:

creatinine (urine) and surface tension

Value Label	Sum	Mean	Std Dev	Sum of Sq	Cases
1. - 40	2136.4000	45.4553	5.4470	1364.7962	47
2. 40 - 80	4290.1000	44.2278	5.0129	2412.3748	97
3. 80 - 120	5481.5000	44.5650	4.4970	2467.1597	123
4. 120 - 160	5103.2000	43.6171	4.2635	2108.5658	117
5. 160 - 200	2463.5000	44.0583	3.5010	723.1458	60
6. 200 - 240	1080.1000	43.2040	4.3679	457.8896	25
7. 240 - 280	484.4000	44.0364	3.5444	125.6255	11
8. 280 - 320	424.3000	47.1444	3.4537	95.4222	9
9. 300 -	228.3000	45.6600	2.2468	20.1920	2
within Groups Total	21871.8000	44.2749	4.4894	9775.1716	494

Analysis of Variance

Source	Sum of Squares	D.F.	Mean Square	F	Sig.
Between Groups	242.4971	8	30.3121	1.5040	0.1531
Within Groups	9775.1716	485	20.1550		

Eta = .1556 Eta Squared = .0242

Figure 2

Mean surface tension depending on Na^+ - levels in urine

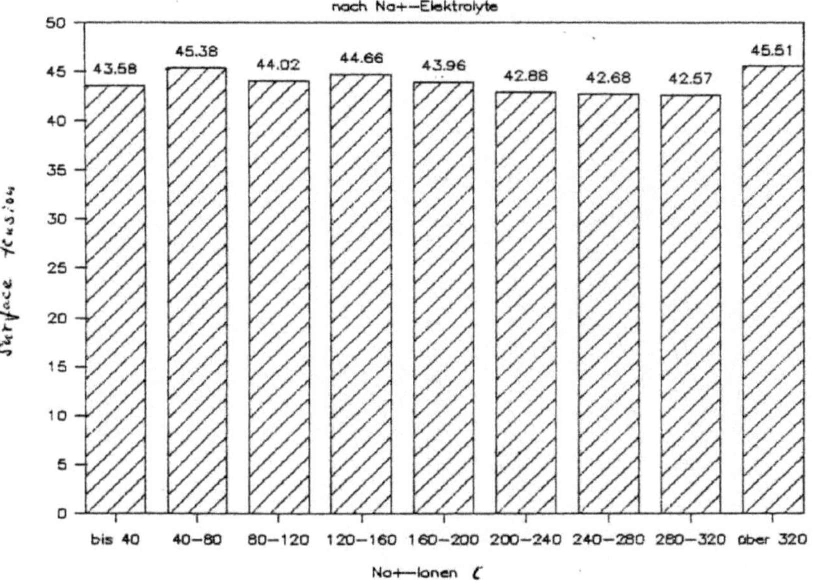

Figure 3

Mean surface tension depending on Ca^{++} - levels in urine

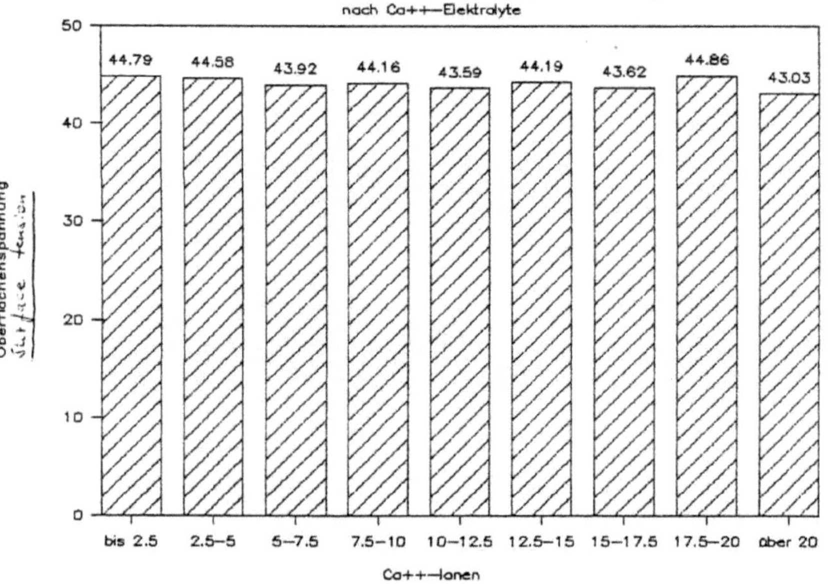

Figure 4

Mean surface tension depending of K^{+}* - levels in urine

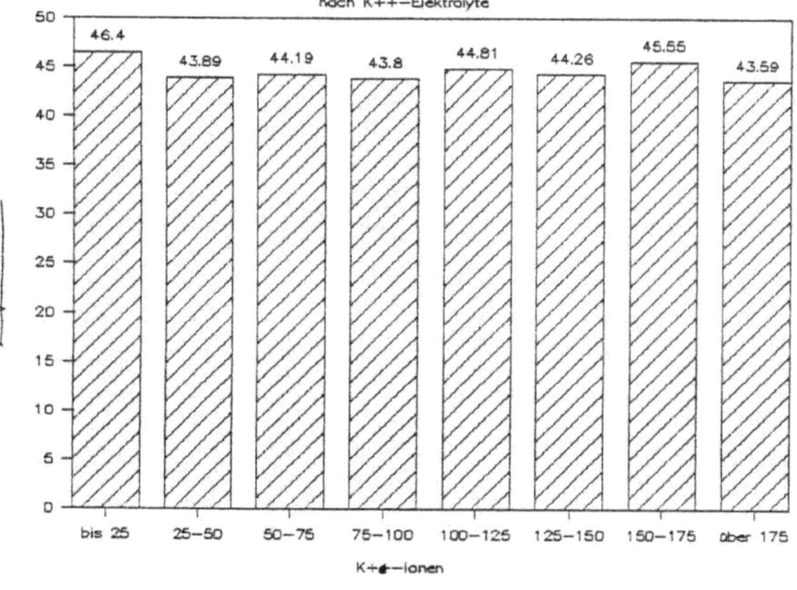

Figure 5

Mean surface tension
given with respect to the pH-value of urine

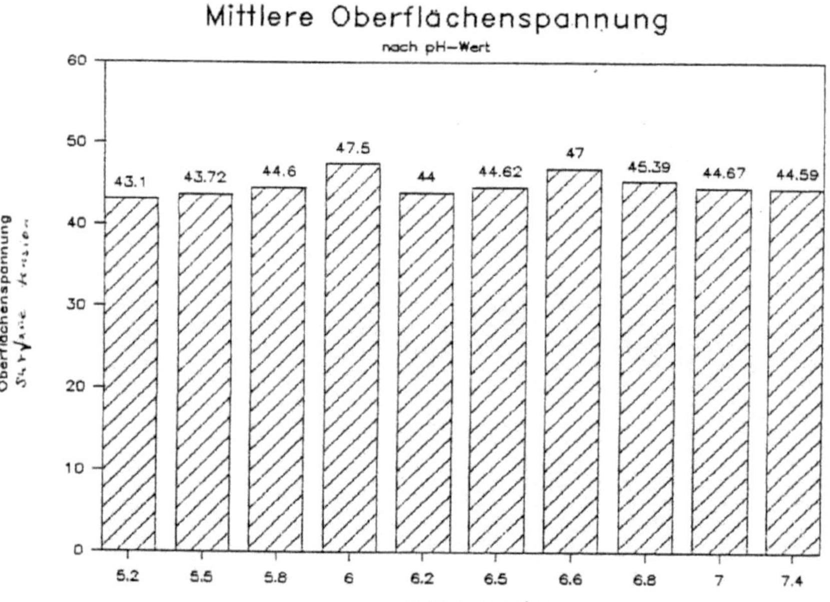

Figure 6

Mean surface tension
given with respect to levels of uric acid in urine

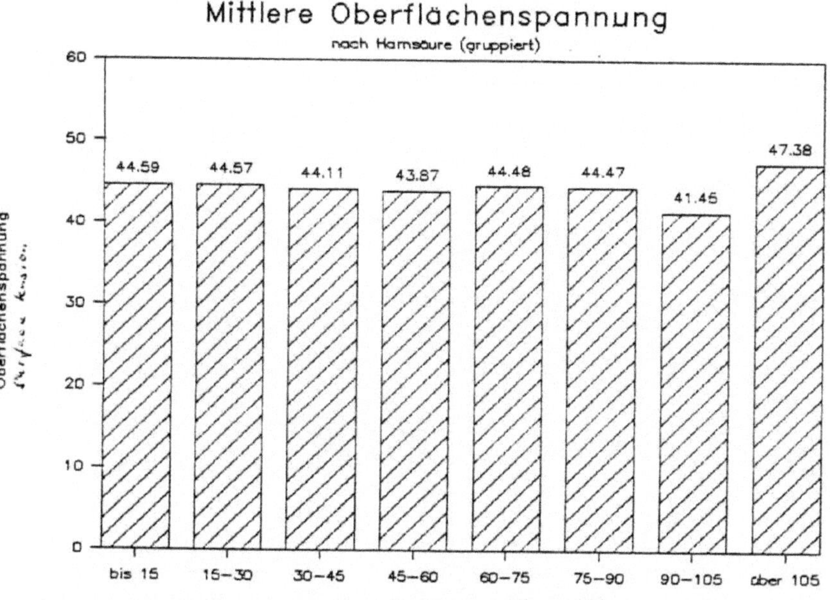

Figure 7

Mean surface tension depending on levels of creatinine in urine

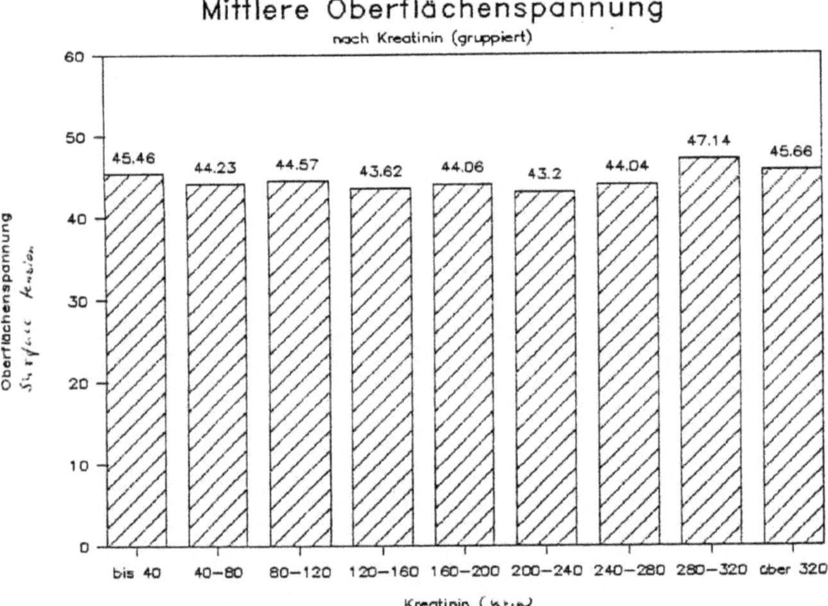

When classifying the data according to the number of leucocytes observed, the quantity of bacteria found, the crystals noted and the STIX-results (testing for blood, protein and glucose in urine; ECURTEST(R) Boehringer Mannheim Corp., W.-Germany) also no special observations with respect to a deviation of the surface tension from the mean value was noted (Fig. 8 through 13, tables No. 8, 9, 10, 11, 12, 13).

Table No. 8

Statistics:

surface tension and number of leucocytes in urine

Value Label	Sum	Mean	Std Dev	Sum of Sq	Cases
1. none	12080.0000	44.2491	4.5767	5697.3623	273
2. up to 5	2583.1000	45.3175	4.9963	1397.9425	57
3. up to 10	1183.8000	45.5308	3.9893	397.8554	26
4. up to 20	776.0000	43.1111	4.8017	391.9578	18
5. up to 50	1568.2000	43.5611	4.7245	781.2456	36
6. up to 100	972.4000	44.2000	3.2712	224.7200	22
7. up to 100	2750.3000	43.6556	3.9382	961.5956	63
within Groups Total	21913.8000	44.2703	4.4933	9852.6790	495

Analysis of Variance

Source	Sum of Squares	D.F.	Mean Square	F	Sig.
Between Groups	170.1545	6	28.3591	1.4046	.2109
Within Groups	9852.6790	488	20.1899		

Eta = .1303 Eta Squared = .0170

Table No. 9

Statistics:

surface tension and quantity of bacteria found in urine

Value Label	Sum	Mean	Std Dev	Sum of Sq	Cases
1. none	20520.6000	44.3210	4.5742	9666.6868	463
2. sporadically	91.7000	45.8500	5.1619	26.6450	2
3. a few	186.3000	46.5750	4.6864	65.8875	4
4. lots of	41.5000	41.5000	0.0	0.0	1
5. masses of	1033.5000	43.0625	2.7736	176.9363	24
within Groups Total	21873.6000	44.2785	4.5077	9936.1555	494

Analysis of Variance

Source	Sum of Squares	D.F.	Mean Square	F	Sig.
Between Groups	70.0770	4	17.5193	.8622	.4865
Within Groups	9936.1555	489	20.3193		

Eta = .0837 Eta Squared = .0070

Table No. 10

Statistics:

surface tension and chrystals noted in urine

Value Label	Sum	Mean	Std Dev	Sum of Sq	Cases
1. none	20246.3000	44.3998	4.5042	9231.0700	456
2. sporadically	640.8000	42.7200	3.2099	144.2440	15
3. a few	470.4000	42.7636	5.6587	320.2055	11
4. lots of	204.1000	40.8200	2.8805	33.1880	5
5. masses of	352.2000	44.0250	4.8617	165.4550	8
within Groups Total	21913.8000	44.2703	4.4936	9894.1624	495

Analysis of Variance

Source	Sum of Squares	D.F.	Mean Square	F	Sig.
Between Groups	128.6710	4	32.1678	1.5931	.1749
Within Groups	9894.1624	490	20.1922		

Eta = .1133 Eta Squared = .0128

Table No. 11

surface tension and STIX-results (blood/urine)

Value Label	Sum	Mean	Std Dev	Sum of Sq	Cases
1. none	17674.4000	44.4080	4.6338	8524.4943	398
2. 5 - 10	941.5000	42.7955	5.0088	526.8495	22
3. 50	565.4000	43.9423	4.8416	281.2892	13
4. 250	2732.5000	44.0726	3.1997	624.5034	62
within Groups Total	21913.8000	44.2703	4.5033	9957.1364	495

Analysis of Variance

Source	Sum of Squares	D.F.	Mean Square	F	Sig.
Between Groups	65.6970	3	21.8990	1.0799	.3572
Within Groups	9957.1364	491	20.2793		

Eta = .0810 Eta Squared = .0066

Table No. 12

surface tension and STIX-results (protein/urine)

Value Label	Sum	Mean	Std Dev	Sum of Sq	Cases
1. none	17028.3000	44.2294	4.7055	8502.2983	385
2. Sp.	1470.7000	44.5667	4.0286	519.3533	33
3. - 30	2631.1000	43.8517	3.4090	685.6498	60
4. - 100	564.6000	47.0500	4.2652	200.1100	12
5. - 500	219.1000	43.8200	1.3809	7.6280	5
within Groups Total	21913.8000	44.2703	4.4983	9915.0395	495

Analysis of Variance

Source	Sum of Squares	D.F.	Mean Square	F	Sig.
Between Groups	107.7940	4	26.9485	1.3318	.2570
Within Groups	9915.0395	490	20.2348		

Eta = .1037 Eta Squared = .0108

Table No. 13

surface tension and STIX-results (glucose/urine)

Value Label	Sum	Mean	Std Dev	Sum of Sq	Cases
1. [illegible]o	20747.1000	44.3314	4.5614	9716.7283	468
2. 100	955.8000	43.4455	3.2862	226.7745	22
3. 250	43.0000	43.0000	0.0	0.0	1
4. 300	80.9000	40.4500	2.4749	6.1250	2
5. 1000	87.0000	43.5000	4.9497	24.5000	2
within Groups Total	21913.8000	44.2703	4.5117	9974.1278	495

Analysis of Variance

Source	Sum of Squares	D.F.	Mean Square	F	Sig.
Between Groups	48.7056	4	12.1764	.5982	.6641
Within Groups	9974.1278	490	20.3554		

Eta = .0697 Eta Squared = .0049

Figure 8

Mean surface tension according to number of leucocytes in urine

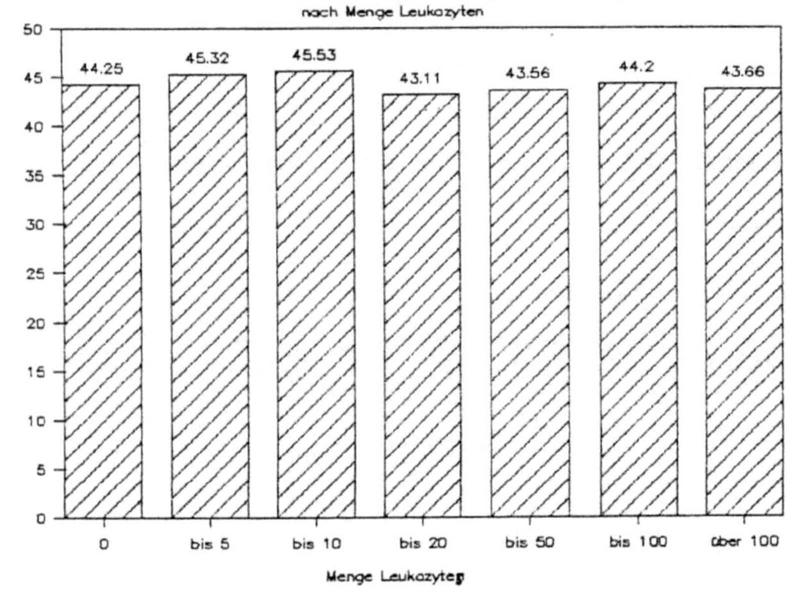

Figure 9

Mean surface tension according to quantity of bacteria found in urine

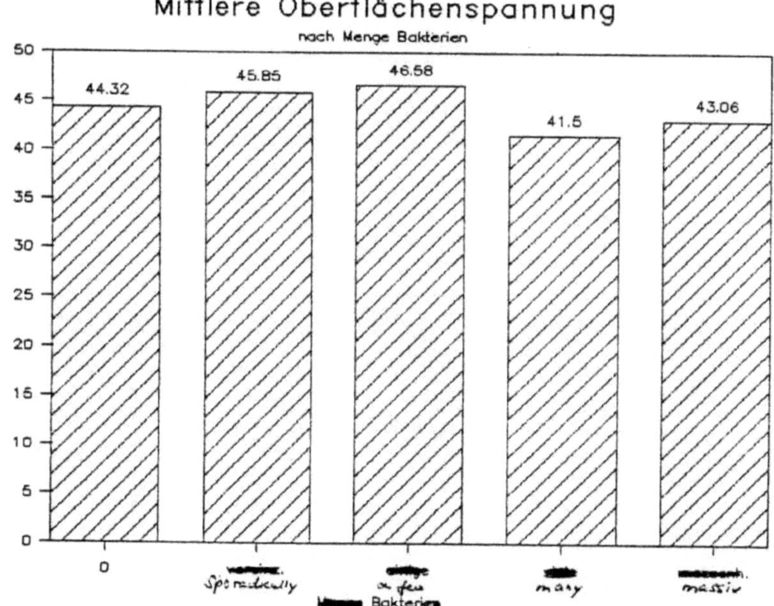

Figure 10

Mean surface tension
given with respect to the crystals noted in urine

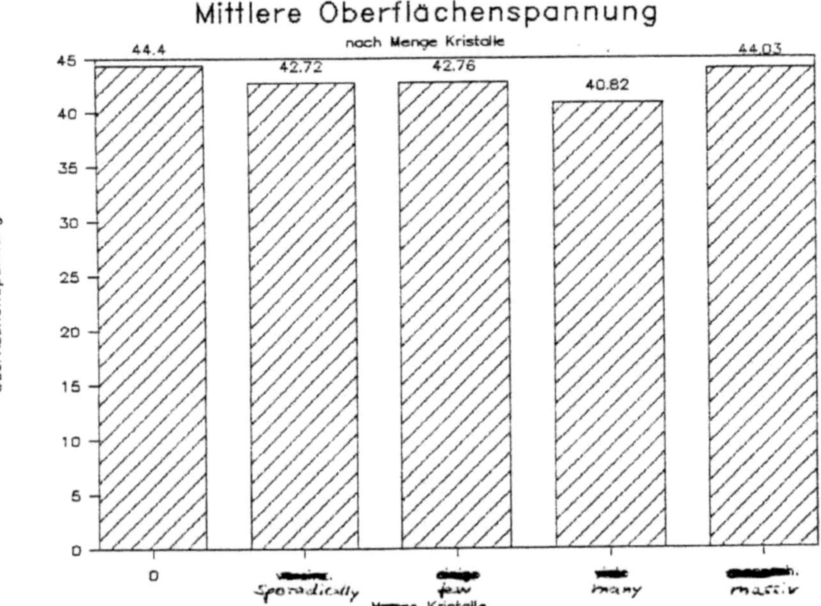

Figure 11

Mean surface tension
based on STIX-results (urine) **(testing for blood)**

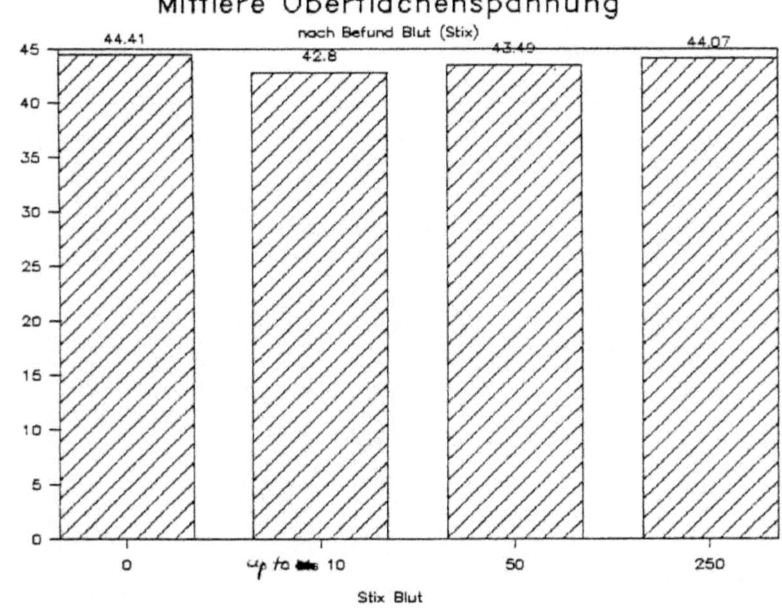

Figure 12

Mean surface tension according to STIX-results (urine) (testing for protein)

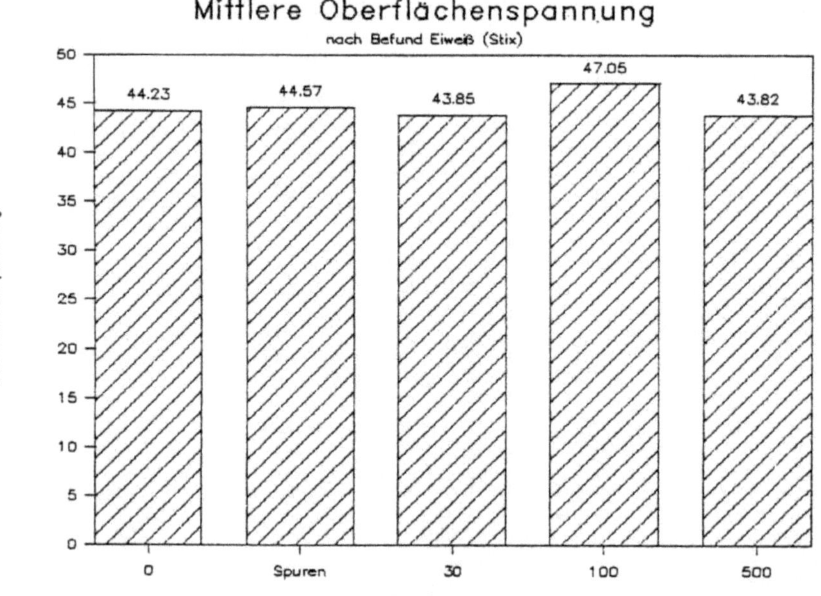

Figure 13

Mean surface tension
according to STIX-results (urine) (testing for glucose)

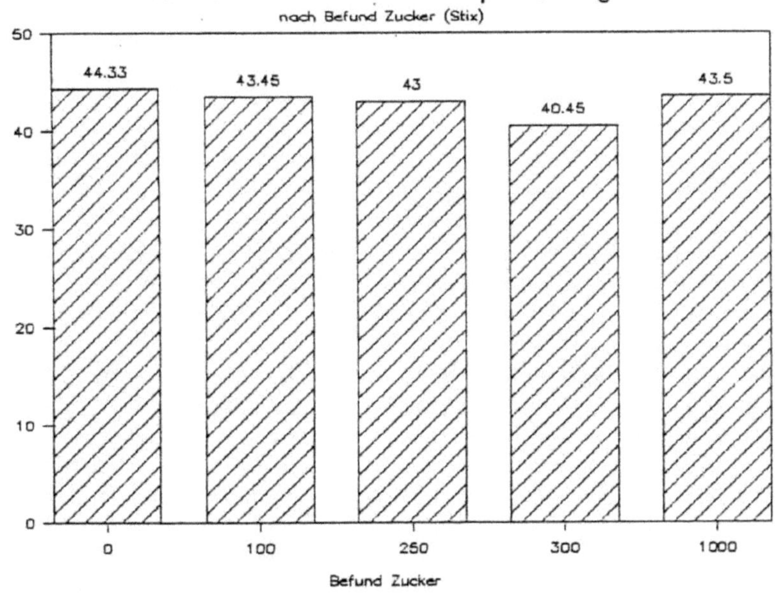

In the scatter plots shown, the concentration of the electrolytes in the urine as referred to the surface tension measured is entered, respectively. From the shape of the scatter plots (a number n signifying n dots at the particular place), which strongly resembles the bell shaped contour of a gaussian distribution, complete independence of the two variables can be deduced (Fig. 14 - 16).

Figure 14

Scatter plot of surface tension (ordinate) and Na^+ - levels (urine) (abscissa)

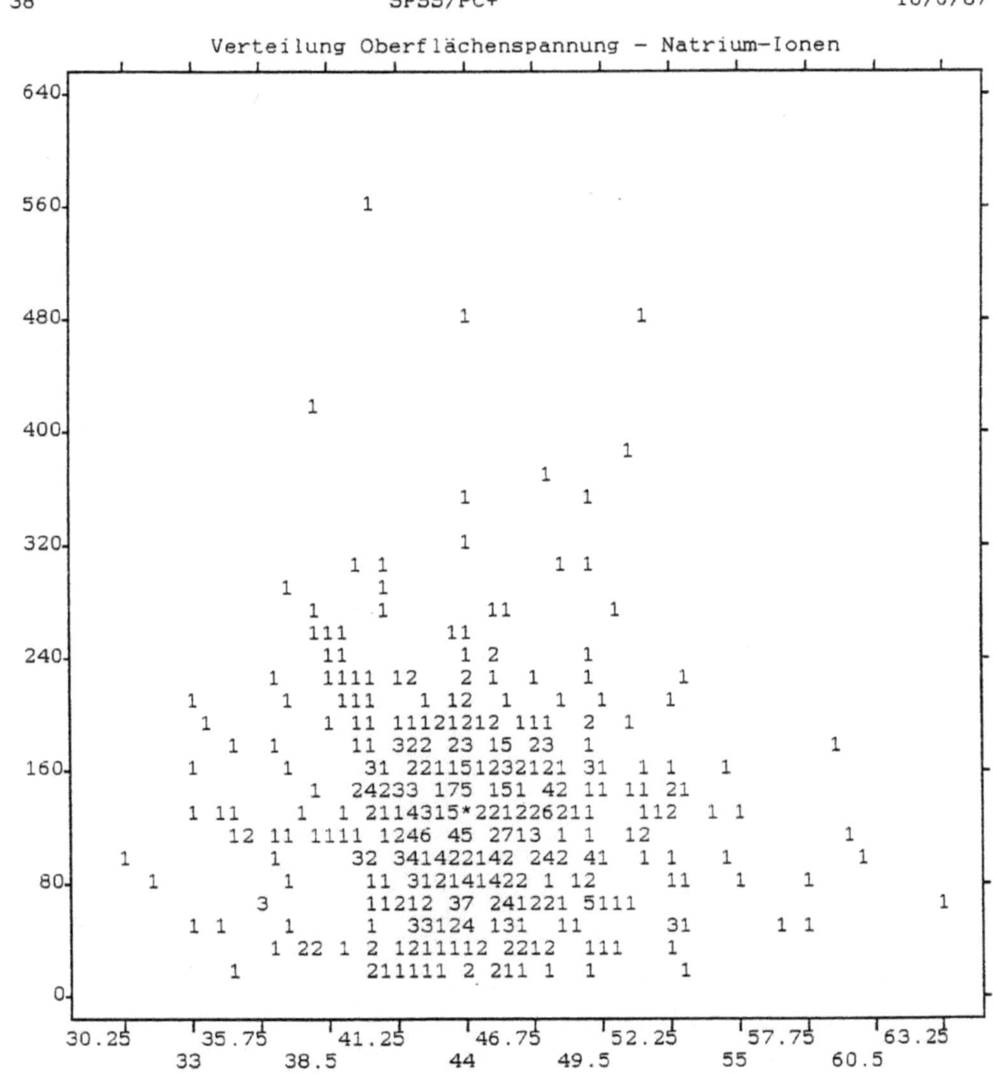

Figure 15

Scatter plot of surface tension (ordinate) and K+ - levels (urine) (abscissa)

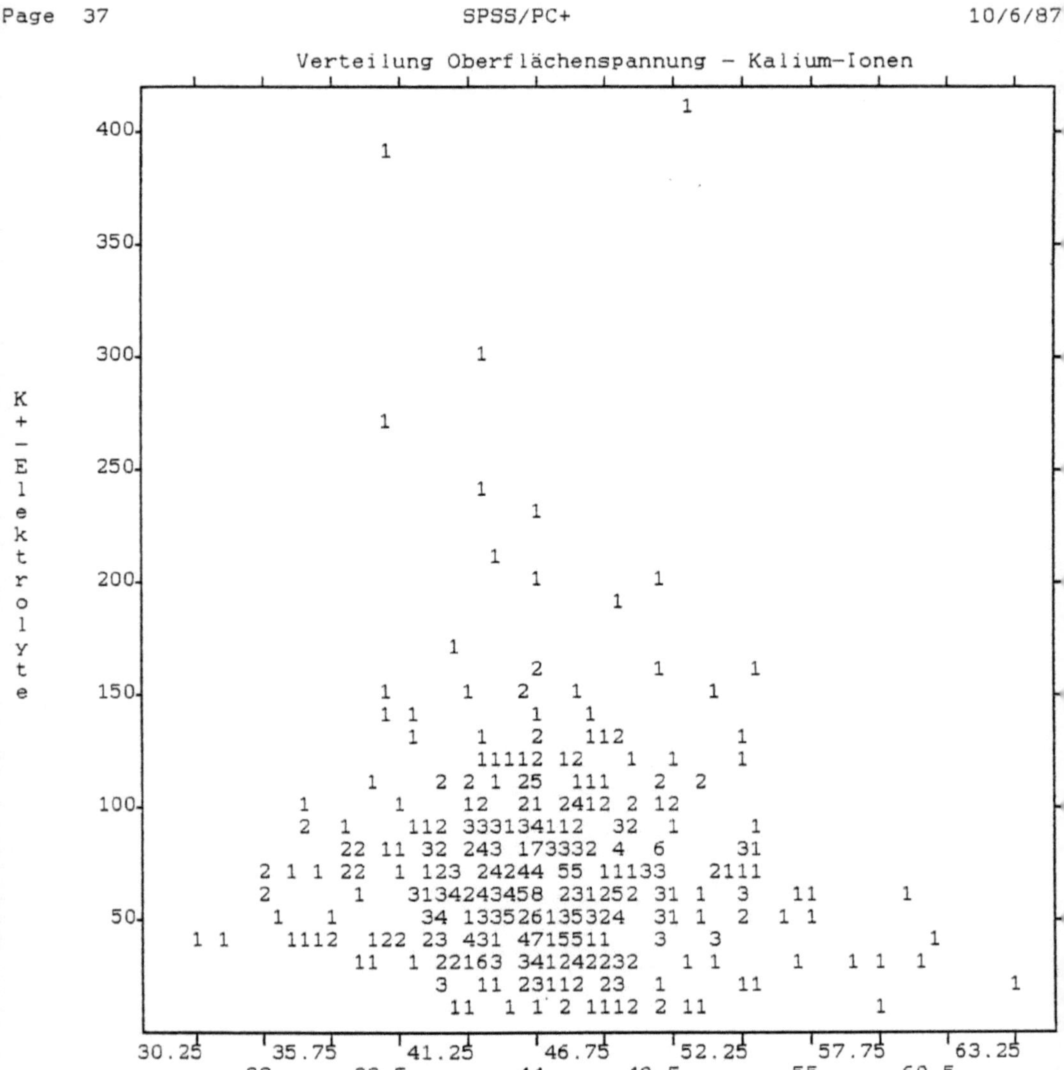

494 cases plotted.

Figure 16

Scatter plot of surface tension (ordinate) and Ca^{++} - levels (urine) (abscissa)

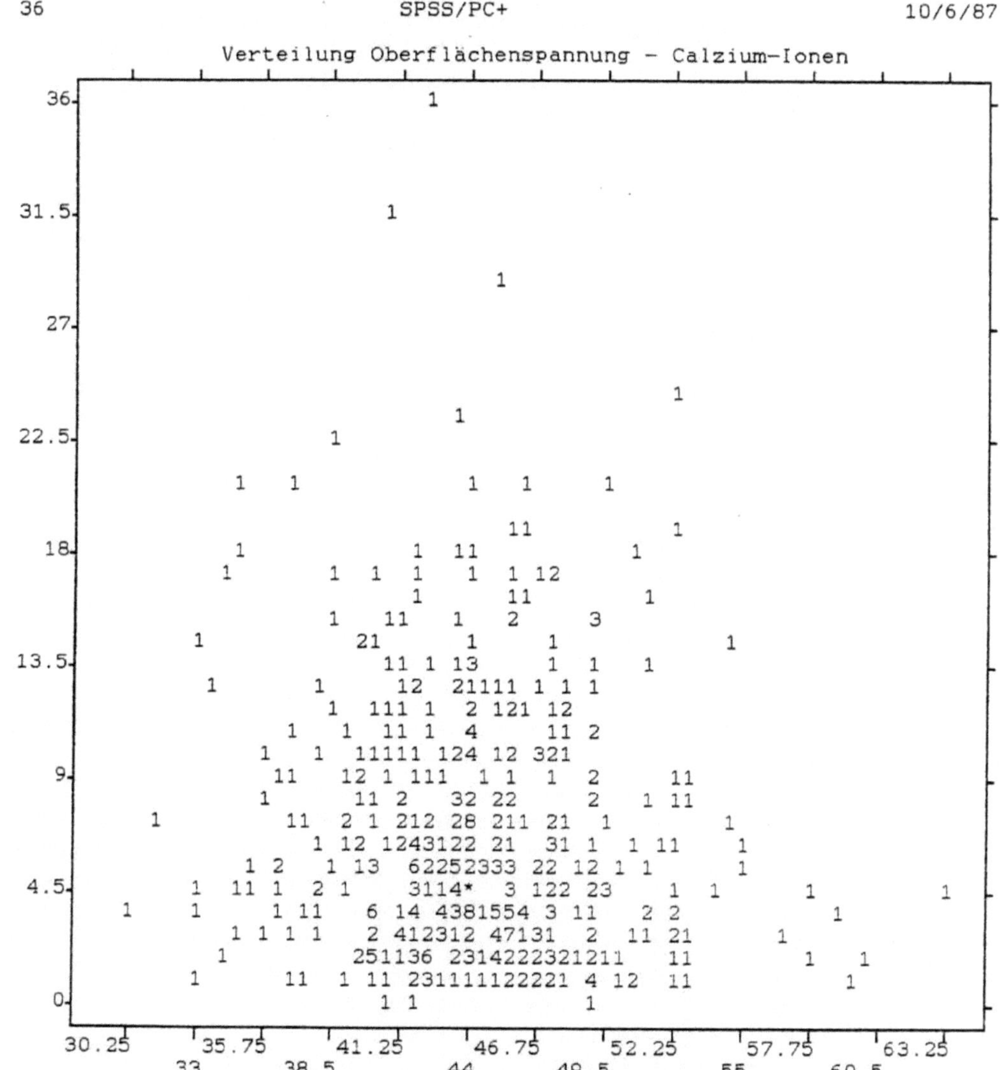

In the investigation of the mean surface tension, as referred to the quantity of erythrocytes (Fig. 17) and epithelial cells counted (Fig 18), significant group differences could be secured by means of variance analysis, but these differences should have no importance. As shown in the figures, the mean surface tensions observed do not rise or fall systematically with the number of erythrocytes counted, resp. with the quantity of epithelial cells observed. Tables No. 14 and 15 give the statistics:

Table No. 14

surface tension and number of erythrocytes(urine)

Value Label	Sum	Mean	Std Dev	Sum of Sq	Cases
1. none	18381.1000	44.1853	4.5123	8449.6206	416
2. up to 5	735.4000	45.9625	4.7279	335.2975	16
2. up to 10	298.8000	49.8000	5.3602	143.6600	6
3. up to 20	242.9000	40.4833	6.0635	183.8283	6
4. up to 50	1096.6000	43.8640	3.7813	343.1576	25
5. up to 100	218.0000	43.6000	2.4280	23.5800	5
6. more than 100	941.0000	44.8095	3.2625	212.8781	21
within Groups Total	21913.8000	44.2703	4.4565	9692.0221	495

Analysis of Variance

Source	Sum of Squares	D.F.	Mean Square	F	Sig.
Between Groups	330.8114	6	55.1352	2.7761	.0116
Within Groups	9692.0221	488	19.8607		

Eta = .1817 Eta Squared = .0330

Table No. 15

surface tension and number of epithelial cells(urine)

Value Label	Sum	Mean	Std Dev	Sum of Sq	Cases
1. none	19916.8000	44.4571	4.3696	8534.9171	448
2. sporadically	215.4000	43.0800	5.5342	122.5080	5
3. a few	961.5000	41.8043	5.8653	756.8496	23
4. lots of	689.8000	43.1125	4.5894	315.9375	16
5. masses of	81.2000	40.6000	7.6368	58.3200	2
within Groups Total	21864.7000	44.2605	4.4741	9788.5322	494

Analysis of Variance

Source	Sum of Squares	D.F.	Mean Square	F	Sig.
Between Groups	210.9281	4	52.7320	2.6343	.0335
Within Groups	9788.5322	489	20.0174		

Eta = .0142 Eta Squared = .0002

Figure 17

Mean surface tension
according to number of erythrocytes in urine

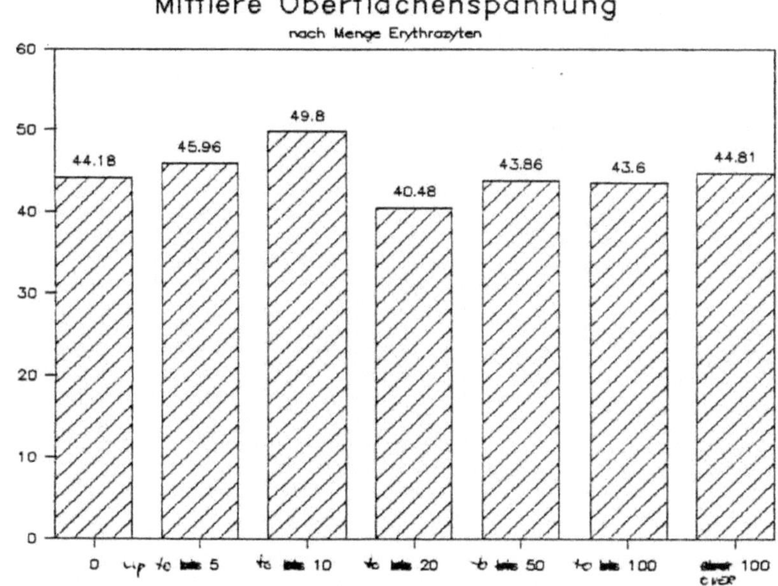

Figure 18

Mean surface tension according to number of epithelial cells

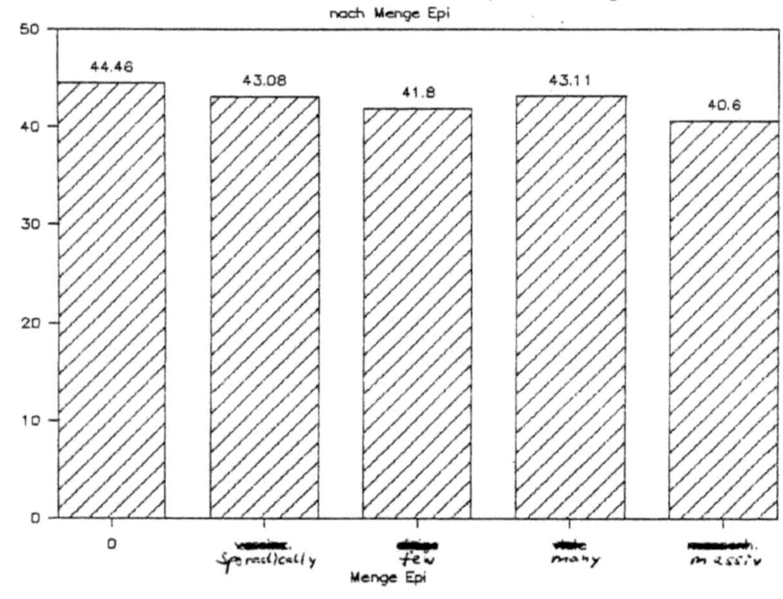

Referring the data measured to the various urological disoders, the following observations can be made: Compared with the mean surface tension of the urine of 384 patients without pathological findings at the kidneys of 44.22 nM/m, the mean value of the 7 Patients with shrunk kidneys was the highest, amounting to 47.19 nM/m. The group differences were statistically not significant however (Fig. 19 and table 16).

Table No. 16

surface tension and pathological kidney findings

Value Label	Sum	Mean	Std Dev	Sum of Sq	Cases
1. no findings	16980.0000	44.2188	4.6386	8240.9850	384
2. kidney tumor	54.2000	54.2000	0.0	0.0	1
3. chron. PN	2178.7000	43.5740	3.3743	557.8962	50
4. acute PN	768.9000	45.2294	3.7696	227.3553	17
5. tuberculosis	47.0000	47.0000	0.0	0.0	1
6. renal shrinkage	330.3000	47.1857	4.0622	99.0086	7
7. renal insufficiency	707.1000	44.1938	3.2146	155.0094	16
8. gout kidneye	92.5000	46.2500	18.7383	351.1250	2
9. renal cyst	755.1000	44.4176	3.3233	176.7047	17
within Groups Total	21913.8000	44.2703	4.4924	9808.0841	495

Analysis of Variance

Source	Sum of Squares	D.F.	Mean Square	F	Sig.
Between Groups	214.7493	8	26.8437	1.3301	.2260
Within Groups	9808.0841	486	20.1812		

Eta = .1464 Eta Squared = .0214

The correlations between diseases of the kidneys and the surface tension of the urine, classified according to the sex of the patients, are listed in Table No. 18.

Compared with a value of 44.49 nM/m for 408 patients without vesical disturbances, the mean surface tension of the urine in patients with chronical cystitis (41.32 nM/m) and particularly in patients suffering from cystitis induced by ionizing radiation (40.63 nM/m) was clearly lower. When variance analysis was performed, the group differences were statistically highly significant ($p = 0.0014$), see also Fig. 20 and table 17.

Table No. 17

surface tension and cystoscopic findings

Value Label	Sum	Mean	Std Dev	Sum of Sq	Cases
1. no findings	18153.4000	44.4936	4.4279	7979.6634	408
2. carcinoma of the bladder	864.7000	45.5105	5.0714	462.9379	19
3. chronic cystitis	1239.7000	41.3233	3.4357	324.3137	30
4. acute cystitis	981.9000	44.6318	4.5777	440.0677	22
5. radiation cystitis	121.9000	40.6333	1.1930	2.8467	3
6. disturbed micturition	552.2000	42.4769	5.7773	400.5231	13
within Groups Total	21913.8000	44.2703	4.4373	9628.3525	495

Analysis of Variance

Source	Sum of Squares	D.F.	Mean Square	F	Sig.
Between Groups	394.4810	5	78.8962	4.0069	.0014
Within Groups	9628.3525	489	19.6899		

Eta = .1984 Eta Squared = .0394

Table No. 18

Correlation between deseases of the kidney and surface tension of urine - values given for females and males

SURFACE TENSION	SEX	
	female	male
no urological disorder	112	272
mean	43.4	44.2
SD	7.5	4.2
kidney tumor	0	1
mean	.	54.2
SD	.	0.0
chronic PN	43	7
mean	43.7	42.7
SD	3.5	2.1
acute PN	13	4
mean	45.4	44.6
SD	4.3	1.2
tuberculosis	1	0
mean	47.0	.
SD	0.0	.
renal shrinking	6	1
mean	46.6	50.0
SD	4.2	0.0
renal insufficiency	8	8
mean	44.3	44.1
SD	3.9	2.6
gout kidney	1	1
mean	59.5	33.0
SD		
renal cyst	6	11
mean	43.3	45.0
SD	5.2	1.7

Figure 19

Mean surface tension
according to pathological kidney findings

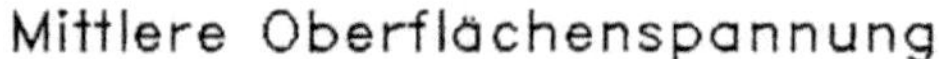

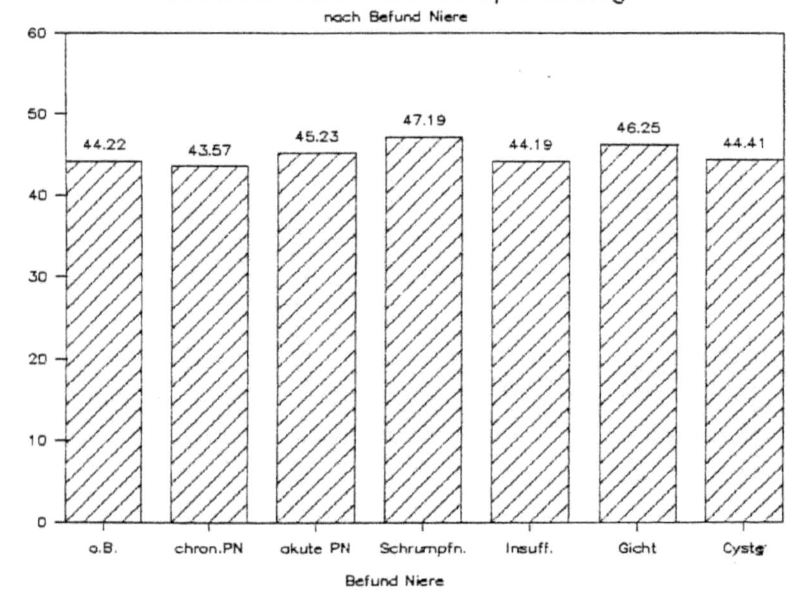

o.B. = no urologic findings
Schrumpfn. = renal shrinking
insuff. = renal insufficiency
Gicht . = gout
Cyste = renal cyst

Figure 20

Mean surface tension according to cystoscopic findings

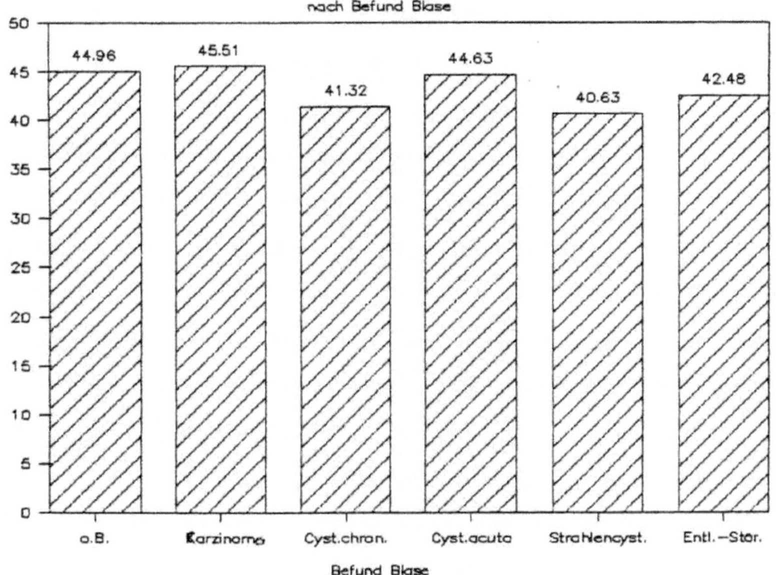

o.B.	=	**no cystiscopic findings**
Karzinom	=	**carcinoma of the bladder**
Strahlencyst.	=	**radiation cystitis**
Entl.-Stör	=	**disturbed micturition**

During evaluation of the measurements as referred to the findings concerning the urinary tract, outliers were clearly noted in cases with proven presence of stones composed of uric acid. The quite low mean surface tension of the urine of 38.94 nM/m was however by no means significantly different as compared with the other groups (Fig.21 and table 19).

Table No. 19

surface tension and findings in the urinary tract

Value Label	Sum	Mean	Std Dev	Sum of Sq	Cases
1. no findings	16435.2000	44.2997	4.6197	7896.3900	371
2. infektion	527.5000	43.9583	4.0198	177.7492	12
3. hyperuricemia	2487.7000	44.4232	4.2192	979.0998	56
4. Ca-oxalate stones	2076.2000	44.1745	3.6388	609.0894	47
5. uric acid stones	194.7000	38.9400	5.5640	123.8320	5
6. urethral strikture	192.5000	48.1250	3.2633	31.9475	4
within Groups Total	21913.8000	44.2703	4.4808	9818.1078	495

Analysis of Variance

Source	Sum of Squares	D.F.	Mean Square	F	Sig.
Between Groups	204.7256	5	40.9451	2.0393	.0718
Within Groups	9818.1078	489	20.0779		

Eta = .1429 Eta Squared = .0204

In the course of investigation of various disorders of the prostate gland, no deviations of the surface tension of the urine as compared with patients without abnormal findings at the prostate gland were observed also (Fig 22 and table 20).

Table No. 20

surface tension and prostate findings

Value Label	Sum	Mean	Std Dev	Sum of Sq	Cases
1. no findings	14069.8000	44.1060	4.7019	7030.3387	319
2. carcinoma of the prostate	541.6000	45.1333	3.0173	100.1467	12
3. chronic prostatitis	1143.9000	43.9962	3.4254	293.3296	26
4. acute prostatitis	1170.0000	43.3333	3.5080	319.9600	27
5. adenoma	4720.0000	44.9524	4.5512	2154.2019	105
6. Sphincter-sclerosis	43.2000	43.2000	0.0	0.0	1
7. post TURP	225.3000	45.0600	2.6708	28.5320	5
within Groups Total	21913.8000	44.2703	4.5101	9926.5089	495

Analysis of Variance

Source	Sum of Squares	D.F.	Mean Square	F	Sig.
Between Groups	96.3246	6	16.0541	.7892	. 5786
Within Groups	9926.5089	488	20.3412		

Eta= .0980 Eta Squared = . 0096

Figure 21

Mean surface tension
according to findings concerning to the urinary tract

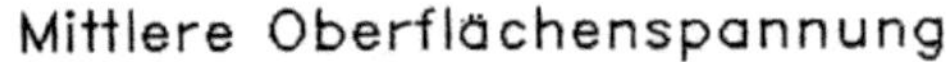

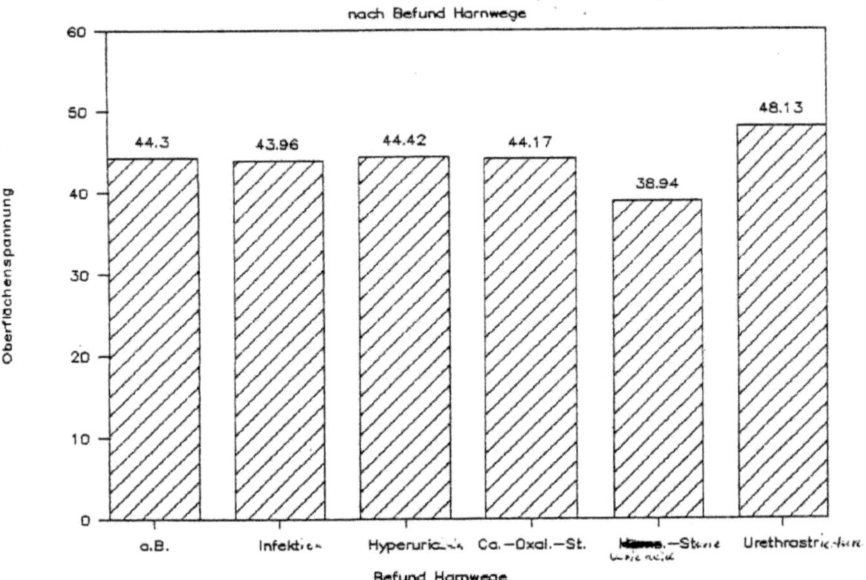

Figure 22

Mean surface tension according to disorders of the prostate gland

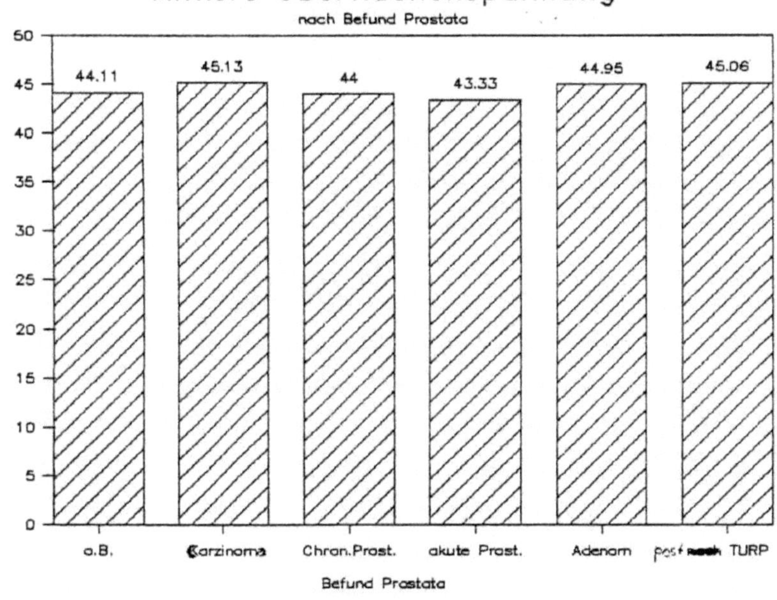

Discussion

The importanceof surface science generally in biology and technology, specially in this subject surface tension and its changes under various conditions in human liquids, was pointed out repeatedly in the past by a large number of authors in all fields of science.

The discrepancies in the results quoted in the literature are fairly large however, not only with respect to the actually measured results, but also regarding the eventual diagnostic, respectivly clinical significance of the obtained data as well as the measuring methods used. As an example I quote the existant data for normal surface tension of human serum,which range from 56.2 nM/m (6) up to 65.0 nM/m (9)

Mottaghy et al. (10) emphasized in 1981 the importance of the temperature and the age of the surfaces on the results of measurement and therefore demanded a standardization of measuring procedures. I therefore measured the fresh urin at an avarage room temperature of 25 degrees Celsius.

The fact,that the values of the surface tension of the urine measured in course of this study ranged approximately around 44 nM/m generally - while in the past a literature result of 64 nM/m is quoted could be attributable to this lack of standardisation or better equipment. Recent data regarding surface tension in urologic out-patients are not obtainable.

No measurements of surface tension of human urin in correlation to various urological disorders as well as in patients with no pathologically clinical findings or case history (14-18) have been carried out so far.

The Question,whether the here measured results of a significantly lower surface tension in the urin of patients suffering from from chronis cystitis or radiation cystitis caused by ionizing post-radiation status due to cancer of either uterus or ovary glands is of any significance or not, remains open. Although one has to bear in mind the higher incidence of carcinoma in situ of the bladder in these patients. Furthermore the extent of the change from 'normal'surface tension in these patients is so far unknown, since sufficient material is missing.

I think these investigastions should soon be carried out in a larger number of patients than I have. They could be done in combinating the measurement of membrane fragments of the urothelium cells,which is a unique cell membrane in man. For example the measurement of the urinary excretion of the Glycosaminglycanes on the urin of patients suffering from carcinoma of the bladder and the surface tension of the urin of these patients should be carried out to recieve more information(17)

The same applies to the electronmicroscopic appaerance - with its different techniqus-. Studies of Bladder cancer patients with reganrds to the surface tension of their urin and the electronmicroscopic findings of their tumors are still missing.

Concisely I think, that the determination of the surface tension in these patients in correlation to other proven methods of inverstigation could be of some help in the future,because urin is easily obtained by non invasive methods and the surface tension measurement is cost-effective.

As a further outline I will carefully assume,that it might gain some acception in the future as an'screening method' in andrology.

References

1. Absolom,D.R., Zingg,W., Policova,Z., Neumann,A.W.: Determination of the Surface Tension of Protein Coated Materials by Means of the Advancing Solidification Front Technique.
Trans Am Soc Artif Intern Organs, Vol 29, (1983)

2. Copley, A.L., King, R.G.: A Survey of Surface Hemorhelogical Experiments on the Inhibition of Fibrinogenin Formation Employing Surface Layers of Fibrinogen Systems with Heparins and other Substances. A Contribution on Antithrombogenic Action.
Thrombosis Research 35, (1984) 237-256

3. Stryer,L.:
Biochemistry
W.H.Freeman and Company, San Francisco,U.S.A.
Third German Edition (1985), Vieweg, Braunschweig,West-Germany

4. Gosling,J.A.:
Atypical muscle cells in the wall of the renal calix and pelvis with a note on their possible significance.
Experientia (Basel,Switzerland) 26 (1970) 769-foll.

5. Gosling,J.A., Dixon,J.S.:
Morphologic evidence that renal calyx and pelvis control ureteric activity in the rabbit.
Am.J.Anat. 130 (1971) 393-foll.

6. Künzel,O.
Ergebn. Inn. Med. Kinderheilkd. 60 (1941), 565-656

7. Loiseleur, J. (1947):
Technique de Laboratoire
Masson et Cie (Editeurs), Libraires del l'Académie de Médicine, Chapitre V, Paris pp. 52-54

8. Masson, D., Diedrich, K., Rehm, G., Stefan, M. u. Schultze-Mosgau, H. (1977):
Geburtshilfe Frauenheilk. 37, 57-63

9. Moser, H.P.:
Elektronenmikroskopische Untersuchungen am Übergangsepithel des menschlichen Nierenbeckens.
Dissertation FU Berlin (1978)

10. Mottaghy, K., Hahn, A.:
Interfacial Tension of Some Biological Fluids: A Comparative Study.
J. Clin. Chem. Clin. Biochem. Vol. 19, (1981) 267-271

11. Mysels, K.J.:
Surface Tension Studies of Bile Salt Association.
Hepatology Vol. 4 (5), (1984) 80-84

12. Schott, H.:
Saturation Adsorption at Interfaces of Surfactant Solution.
Journal of Pharmaceutical Sciences, Vol. 69 No. 7, (1980)

13. Weser, C.:
Die Messung der Grenz- und Oberflächenspannung von Flüssigkeiten - eine Gesamtdarstellung für den Praktiker -
GIT Fachzeitschrift für das Laboratiorium, 24, (1980) 642-648 and 734-742

14. Karlson,P.,Gerok,W.,Groß:
Pathobiochemie
G.-Thieme Verlag, Stuttgart and New York
Second Edition 1982

15. Schneider,H.J. (Editor):
Urolithiasis:Etiology - Diagnosis
Springer-Verlag,Berlin,Heidelberg,New York,Tokyo
1985

16. Schneider,H.J. (Editor)
Urolithiasis: Therapy-Prevention
Springer-Verlag,Berlin,Heidelberg,New York,Tokyo
1986

17. Bichler,K.H., Harzmann,R.:
Das Harnblasenkarzinom
Springer-Verlag,Berlin,Heidelberg,New York,Tokyo
1984

18. Prince,L.M., Sears,D.F.:
Biological horizons in surface science
Academic Press, New York, 1973

Supplement

Compilation of Literature on boundary and surface-tension of nonliquid and liquid materials (with gratitude to Krüss Corp., Hamburg, West-Germany)

Du Noüy, An Apparatus for Measuring Surface Tension. Journal of General Physiology 1, 521, 1919

Du Noüy, The Surface Equilibrium of Colloidal Solutions and the Dimensions of some Colloidal Molecules. Science, 59, 580, 1924.

Du Noüy, The Surface Tension of Colloidal Solutions and the Dimensions of Certain Organic Molecules.Phil.Mag.48,262, 1924.

Du Noüy, Some New Aspects of the Surface Tension of Colloid Solutions, Third National Symposium Monograph 25, 1927

Klopsteg, A Note on the Ring Method of the Measuring Surface Tension.Science 60, 1924.

Du Noüy, An Interfacial Tensiometer for Universal Use.Journ. of General Physiology 7, 625, 1925.

Du Noüy, Surface Equilibris of Colloids. A.C.S. Monograph Series, 1926.

Klopsteg, Surface Tension Measurements by the Ring Method. Science 63, 1926.

Rideal, An Introduction to Surface Chemistry.University press. Cambridge 1926.

Bakker, Kapillarität und Oberflächenspannung, Akadem.Verlagsgesellschaft, Leipzig 1928.

W.D.Harkins and H.F.Jordan,
"a method for the determination of surface and interfacial-tension from the maximum pull on a ring"
J.Amer, Soc.52.2, 1751 (1930)

Hercik, Oberflächenspannung in der Biologie und Medizin, Theodor Steinkopf, Dresden 1933.

Clayton, The Theory of Emulsions and their Technical Treatment. J.A. Churchill, London 1935.

Seelich, Die Komplementbindung als Grenzflächenreaktion. Bioch. Z.286, 396, 1936.

Seelich, Beitrag zur Kenntnis der Kationenwirkung an Grenzflächen von acidoidem Charakter. Koll. Z.85. 268. 1938.

Trillát, Öl und Kohle 14, 177, 1938.

Müller, Über die Schmierung von Otto-Motoren in Kraftfahrzeugen.Bericht der Gemeinschaftstagung der Fachgruppe Brennstoff und Mineralölchemie und der Deutschen Gesellschaft für Mineralölforschung, Frankfurt a.M. 1938.

Seelich, Über einige physikalisch-chemische Bedingungen der Emulsionsbildung und der Emulsionsstabilität.Fette und Seifen 46, 139, 1939.

Seelich, Modellversuche zur biologischen Natrium- und Calciumwirkung. Pflügers Archiv f.d.gesamte Biologie 242,275, 1939.

Seelich, Die Charakterisierung von Ölen durch Bestimmung der Grenzflächenspannung gegen Wasser oder wäßrige Lösungen. Fette und Seifen 41, 15, 1941.

H.Zuidema und C.W.Waters Ind. Engang. chem. Analyt.Edit. (1941) 312-313 Korrekturgleichung für die Grenzflächenspannungen.

Standard Method of Test for Interfacial Tension of Oil against Water by the Ring Method (ASTM Designation:D 971-50 adopted 1950) by the American Standards Association. ASA No.Z.II.64-1950.

H.W.Fox, C.H.Chrisman: "The Ring Method of Measuring Surface Tension for Liquids of high Density and low Surface Tension".
Naval Research Laboratory, Washinton D.C. (2/1951)

Wachs und Heine, Darstellung von Monoglyceriden ungesättigter Fettsäuren mit Hilfe der Molekulardestillation und Untersuchung ihrer emulgierenden Eigenschaften. Fette und Seifen 54. 760, 1952.

Oberflächenspannung und Oberflächenaktivität, Hauben-Weyl, Methoden der organischen Chemie, 4. Aufl. (1955) Bd.III Teil 1.

Kluge,Eicke und Balz, Ein Beitrag zur Prüfung von Zähler-, Uhren- und Feinmechanikölen, Feinwerktechnik 60, 165, 1956.

K.Hintzmann, Eine meßtechnische Methode zur Ermittlung der Grenzflächenkräfte eines hydrophobierten Oberflächenbildes gegenüber Wasser und ihre Beziehungen zum Hydrophobiereffekt. Melliand Textilberichte 41, 3/1960.

J.F.Padday, D.R.Russell: "The Measurement of the Surface Tension of Pure Liquids and Solutions".J.of Colloid Sci. 15, 503-511 (1960)

J.Buchi & X.Perlin, Oberflächenaktivität der Cinchocain-Homologen. Arzneimittelforschung, Editio Cantor KG.11.Jahrgang, 11, 1961 No.9

Oberflächen- und Grenzflächenspannung, Ullmanns Encyklopädie der technischen Chemie, München-Berlin 1961, Band 2/1.

K.Durham: "Surface Activity and Detergency"
London Macmillan & Co. Ltd., New York, St.Martin's Press 1961.

H.Lange: "Oberflächen- und Grenzflächenspannungsmessung" Ullmanns Encyklopädie der techn. Chemie, Band 2/1. 1961.

Dr.sc. techn.G.Anderees, Einfluß der Oberflächenspannung auf den Stoffaustausch zwischen Dampfblasen und Flüssigkeit. Chemie-Ing. Techn.34. 1962, No.9

Führer und Kilb, Zur Meßtechnik der Ober- und Grenzflächenspannung. Ztschr. f.Instrumentenkunde 71, 2, 1963.

G.Marwedel, Zusammenhänge zwischen Oberflächenspannung,Dichte und Viskosität organischer Flüssigkeiten bei gleichen Temperaturen.Farbe und Lack 69, 6, 1963.

Chem.-Ing.Christa Poley und Chem.-Ing.K.Kurzweg, Untersuchungen über Oberflächenstörungen bei Einbrennlacken am Beispiel einer Epoxidharz-Alkydharz-Melaminharz-Kombination, Mitteilung der VEB Lackfabrik Berlin.

Dr.F.van Voorst Vader, Die Stabilität von Emulsionen und Schäumen, Fette-Seifen-Anstrichmittel, 66.Jahrgang No.1, 1964.

A.W.Neumann:"Über die Meßmethodik zur Bestimmung grenzflächenenergetischer Größer"
2.physik.Chem.Neue Folge 41, 1964 S.339-352
2.physik.Chem.Neue Folge 41, 1964 S.71-83.

H.L.Rosano:Study of the Foamability of Solutions Using the Tensiolaminometric Technique" AOCS Vol.45 No.8, 607-610 (1967).

Dipl.Ing.K.Feldkamp, Die Oberflächenspannung wäßriger NaOH- und KOH-Lösungen,Chemie- Ing.Techn.41.Jahrg.1969 No.21.

P.J.Sell, A.W.Neumann:"Oberflächen- und Volumeneigenschaften von Cholesterylestern homologer Fettsäuren". Zeitschrift für Physikalische Chemie Bd.65, S.13-18 (1969)

R.Hensch:"Eine experimentelle Methode zur Bestimmung des HLB-Wertes vonTensiden".
Kolloid-Zeitschrift + Zeitschrift für Polymere Vol.236 No.1, 31-38 (1970)

H.Linde:"Fortschritte auf dem Gebiet der Grenzflächendynamik". Chem.Techn.Vol.22 No.3 (3/1970)

A.W.Neumann: "Bedeutung und Bestimmung grenzflächenenergetischer Größen im Hinblick auf technische Fragestellungen" Chemie, Ingenieur, Technik (15/1970) S.969-1016.

M.J.Schwager, H.M.Rostek: "Automatische Apparatur zur Messung der Oberflächenspannung nach der Wilhelmy-Methode". Chem.Ing.Techn.43 No.19 (1971).

P.J.Cram, J.M.Haynes: "The Influence of the Contact Angle on Surface Tension Measurements by the Ring Detachment Method"
Journal of Colloid and Interface Science. Vol.35, No.4 April 1971.

Renato Cini, Giuseppe Loglio and Augusto Ficalbi: "Temperature Dependence of the Surface Tension of Water by the Equilibrium Ring Method". Colloid & Interface Sci. Vol.41, No.2 (Nov.1972).

G.Koerner, G.Rossmy and G.Sänger:"Zur Lösung von Grenzflächenproblemen"
Goldschmidt informiert, 2/1974 No.29.

H.L.Rosano: "Microemulsions"
J.Soc.Cosmet. Chem. 25, 609-619 (11/1974)

H.Brüschweiler:"Eigenschaften und biologisches Abbauverhalten von grenzflächenaktiven Verbindungen"
Chimia 29, No.1 (1975)

C.Huh and S.G.Mason:" A rigorous theory of ring tensiometry". Colloid Polymer Sci.253, 566-580 (1975).

D.N.Furlong, S.Hartland: "Wall Effect in the Determination of Surface Tension using a Wilhelmy Plate", VII International Congress on Surface Activity,Moscow Sept.1976.

M.Burkowsky, C.Marx:"Use of the Spinning Drop Interfacial-Tensiometer for Evaluation of Surfactants for low Tension Flooding - An Experience Report". Oil Gas-European Magazin (2/77).

R.Finzel, F.W.Seemann:"Korrekturtabellen für das Ringverfahren zur Messung der Oberflächenspannung" PTB-Mitteilungen 87, 295-300 (4/1977).

F.Bauer, K.J.Hüttinger:"Einfluß von Tensiden auf Grenzflächenspannung und Stoffübergang in flüssigen Zweiphasensystemen". Chem.Ing.Tech.50, No.6 (1978).

YOUR KNOWLEDGE HAS VALUE

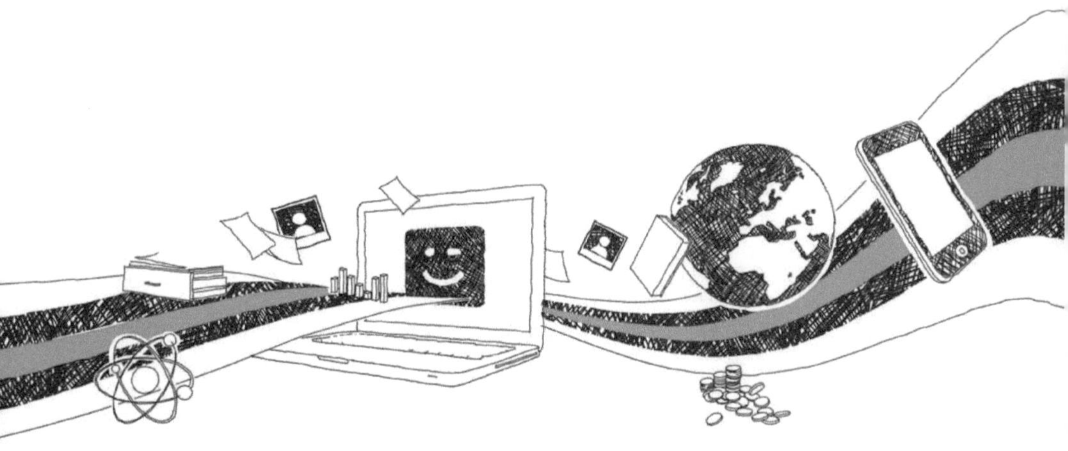

- We will publish your bachelor's and master's thesis, essays and papers
- Your own eBook and book - sold worldwide in all relevant shops
- Earn money with each sale

Upload your text at www.GRIN.com and publish for free

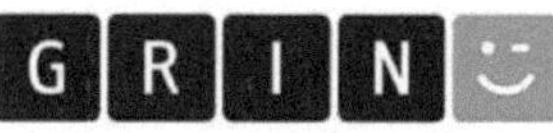